Duphas Pregnancy

How Essential and Safe Is It?

Asharani Sah

Duphaston in Pregnancy

How Essential and Safe Is It?

Author: Asharani Sah
Published by: Self-Published

First Edition (Paperback Format)

Copyright © 2025 Asharani Sah

All rights reserved. No part of this publication may be reproduced, stored in a retrieval system, or transmitted in any form or by any means—electronic, mechanical, photocopying, recording, or otherwise—without the author's prior written permission.

ISBN: 978-93-342-5301-6

Dedication

To Lord Shri Ramakrishna

Preface

In the ever-evolving field of obstetrics and gynaecology, the use of hormonal therapies remains a cornerstone of patient care. Among these, **dydrogesterone**—marketed as Duphaston 10mg—has emerged as a widely prescribed progestogen, particularly in the management of pregnancy-related conditions such as threatened miscarriage, recurrent pregnancy loss, and luteal phase support in assisted reproductive technology (ART). Yet, despite its widespread use, questions persist: *Is dydrogesterone truly safe during pregnancy? Is it always necessary? And how does it compare to other progestogens in terms of efficacy and risk?*

This book, *"Dydrogesterone (Duphaston) in Pregnancy: How Essential and Safe Is It?"*, was born out of a need to address these questions with clarity, depth, and evidence-based rigor. As healthcare professionals, our primary responsibility is to our patients, and making informed decisions about their care requires a thorough understanding of the medications we prescribe. This guide aims to provide you with precisely that—a comprehensive, clinically relevant resource that bridges the gap between research and practice.

Why This Book?

Over the years, dydrogesterone has been the subject of numerous studies, clinical trials, and debates. While some hail it as a safe and effective option for progesterone support, others urge caution, citing potential risks and the need for further research. As practitioners, we are often left navigating this complex landscape, balancing the benefits of treatment against the potential for adverse outcomes.

What to Expect

Inside, you will find:

- A detailed exploration of dydrogesterone's **mechanism of action, pharmacokinetics,** and **pharmacodynamics**.
- Evidence-based insights into its **clinical applications**, from threatened miscarriage to luteal phase support and beyond.
- A critical analysis of its **safety profile**, including maternal and foetal outcomes, potential risks, and contraindications.
- Practical guidance on **dosage adjustments, patient monitoring,** and **managing adverse effects**.
- Real-world **case studies** and **clinical scenarios** to help you apply the evidence in your practice.

A Note on Perspective

This book is not intended to advocate for or against the use of dydrogesterone. Rather, it seeks to present the facts as they are, empowering you to make informed, patient-centred decisions. We recognize that every patient is unique, and what works for one may not work for another. Our goal is to equip you with the knowledge and tools to tailor your approach to each individual's needs.

A Final Word

As you delve into the pages of this book, we hope it serves not only as a source of knowledge but also as a catalyst for reflection and discussion. Medicine is a collaborative endeavour, and we invite you to join the conversation, challenge assumptions, and continue pushing the boundaries of what we know.

Thank you for your commitment to excellence in patient care. We trust that this book will be a valuable addition to your practice and a resource you turn to time and again.

Warm regards,

Asharani Sah

--------Disclaimer----------

This book is intended for educational purposes only and is not a substitute for professional medical advice. Always consult a qualified healthcare provider before taking any medication, including Duphaston (dydrogesterone).

While efforts have been made to ensure the accuracy of the information, medical knowledge is constantly evolving. The content of this book should not be considered exhaustive or relied upon solely for medical decisions.

The author, Asharani Sah, does not endorse any specific tests, physicians, products, or procedures mentioned in this book.

Table of Content

Chapter 1

Introduction to Dydrogesterone............01

The history and development of dydrogesterone (Duphaston)

Why is dydrogesterone prescribed? Understanding its significance in reproductive medicine.

Chapter 2

Pharmacological Profile of Dydrogesterone..7

Mechanism of action: How does Duphaston work in the body?

Pharmacokinetics: Absorption, metabolism, and excretion of dydrogesterone

Comparison with other progestogens – Is Duphaston superior to micronized progesterone?

Chapter 3

Clinical Indications for Dydrogesterone 16

Threatened and habitual miscarriage: Can dydrogesterone prevent pregnancy loss?

Luteal support in ART: Role of dydrogesterone in IVF and assisted reproduction

Infertility due to luteal insufficiency: How does Duphaston improve conception rates?

Other uses in gynaecology: Dysmenorrhea, endometriosis, irregular cycles, and more.

Chapter 4

Safety and Efficacy in Pregnancy...........21

Latest clinical trials & research studies (including LOTUS I & II trials)

Maternal safety profile and foetal outcomes

Risk of congenital anomalies (e.g., hypospadias) – What does the data suggest?

Chapter 5

Dosage and Administration Guidelines..24

Recommended dosage for different conditions

Adjustments based on clinical response

Special populations: Use in adolescents, elderly, and high-risk pregnancies

Chapter 6

Contraindications and Precautions.........28

When NOT to prescribe dydrogesterone

Risks in patients with liver disease, porphyria, or hormone-dependent cancers

Addressing lactose intolerance and excipient-related concerns

Chapter 7

Adverse Effects and Risk Management...31

Common Side Effects

Serious Adverse Reactions

Overdose management and emergency protocols

Chapter 8

Dydrogesterone in Hormone Replacement Therapy (HRT)..35

Role in menopausal therapy: Preventing oestrogen-induced endometrial hyperplasia

Breast cancer risks and mammographic density concerns

Venous thromboembolism and cardiovascular considerations

Chapter 9

Drug Interactions 37

Impact of CYP450 enzyme interactions: Effect of anticonvulsants, rifampicin, and other drugs.

Herbal supplements and alternative therapies: Can they interfere with dydrogesterone metabolism?

Chapter 10

Special Populations and Considerations ..39

Use in adolescents: Is dydrogesterone safe for young women?

Pregnancy and lactation: Can Duphaston be continued postpartum?

Long-term safety in elderly patients

Chapter 11

Clinical Case Studies and Practical Insights.............43

Real-world applications of dydrogesterone in managing pregnancy complications

How to optimize treatment in recurrent miscarriage and IVF patients

Guidance on handling breakthrough bleeding and HRT challenges

Chapter 12: Global Guidelines and Expert Consensus 47

International recommendations on dydrogesterone use

How does Duphaston compare to micronized progesterone in global clinical practice?

Expert opinions on safety, efficacy, and best

Chapter 13: Future Research and Emerging Trends .. 50

Ongoing clinical trials on dydrogesterone

Potential new indications for this synthetic progestogen

Advancements in progesterone therapy and personalized medicine

Chapter 14: Conclusion and Key Takeaways 53

Summary of evidence and clinical guidelines

Final recommendations for medical practitioners

Future role of dydrogesterone in modern obstetrics and gynaecology

Chapter 1:
Introduction to Dydrogesterone

For doctors and medical paramedics, understanding the history of dydrogesterone is more than an academic exercise—it provides a foundation for appreciating its clinical value. The development of dydrogesterone reflects decades of scientific innovation, rigorous testing, and a commitment to improving patient outcomes. As we continue to refine its use and explore new applications, this historical perspective reminds us of the importance of evidence-based practice and the ongoing pursuit of excellence in patient care.

The History and Development of Dydrogesterone

Progesterone is an essential hormone in **pregnancy maintenance, menstrual regulation, and hormone therapy**. However, due to the **poor oral bioavailability of natural progesterone**, researchers sought to develop **synthetic progestogens** that could be used effectively in clinical practice. **Dydrogesterone (Duphaston)** represents a major advancement in this effort, offering **high oral bioavailability, strong progestogenic activity, and minimal side effects**.

Chronological Development of Progestogens and the Need for Dydrogesterone

1. Discovery of Natural Progesterone (1929-1934)

The isolation of natural progesterone from animal ovaries marked the beginning of hormonal therapy. However, its poor oral bioavailability and rapid metabolism limited its clinical use. Researchers sought synthetic alternatives that could mimic its effects more effectively.

2. First-Generation Progestins (1950s–1960s) - Norethisterone and Medroxyprogesterone Acetate (MPA)

These early synthetic progestogens were developed to address the limitations of natural progesterone. However, they often exhibited androgenic or estrogenic side effects, which restricted their use in certain patient populations.

3. Second-Generation Progestins (1960s–1970s) – The Birth of Dydrogesterone (Duphaston)

Dydrogesterone was developed to overcome the limitations of earlier progestogens. Its unique **retrosteroidal configuration** allowed it to bind selectively to progesterone receptors without estrogenic, androgenic, or corticoid activity. This made it a safer and more targeted option for treating progesterone deficiency.

4. Third-Generation and Beyond (1980s–Present) – Micronized Progesterone and Further Refinements

In the **1980s and 1990s**, micronized progesterone was introduced to enhance the **oral bioavailability of natural progesterone**, offering a more physiologically similar alternative to synthetic progestins. While it remains widely used today, it still requires **higher doses**, is associated with **gastrointestinal side effects**, and lacks the **convenience and targeted selectivity** of dydrogesterone. In later years, newer progestins such as **drospirenone and dienogest** were developed primarily for **contraceptive and gynecological applications**; however, they do not replace dydrogesterone's **unique role in pregnancy support and hormone replacement therapy (HRT),** where selective progesterone receptor activation is crucial.

Development of Progestogens

Discovery of Natural Progesterone

The isolation of natural progesterone from animal ovaries marked the beginning of hormonal therapy.

First-Generation Progestins

Synthetic progestogens like Norethisterone and MPA were developed but had significant side effects.

Second-Generation Progestins

Dydrogesterone was developed to overcome the limitations of earlier progestogens.

Third-Generation and Beyond

Micronized progesterone and other progestins were developed, but dydrogesterone remains unique in its role.

The Introduction of Dydrogesterone into Clinical Practice

After its synthesis in the early **1960s**, dydrogesterone was introduced into **clinical use across Europe and Asia** and gained rapid acceptance due to its **superior safety and tolerability profile**.
Key Clinical Applications of Dydrogesterone:

- **Pregnancy Support** – Used for **threatened and recurrent miscarriage**, luteal phase insufficiency, and luteal support in **assisted reproductive technologies (ART)**.

- **Gynecological Disorders** – Effective in **dysmenorrhea, endometriosis, secondary amenorrhea, irregular cycles, and dysfunctional uterine bleeding**.

- **Hormone Replacement Therapy (HRT)** – Provides **endometrial protection** against estrogen-induced hyperplasia in menopausal women.

The drug quickly became **one of the most widely prescribed progestogens worldwide** due to its **efficacy, excellent safety profile, and superior tolerability compared to older synthetic progestins**.

Dydrogesterone vs. Other Progestogens: A Key Advancement

Before dydrogesterone, synthetic progestogens like **norethisterone and medroxyprogesterone acetate (MPA)** were commonly used. However, these **older progestins** had **strong androgenic effects, altered lipid metabolism, and an increased risk of cardiovascular side effects**.

Dydrogesterone was **a breakthrough** because it:

☑ **Lacks androgenic, estrogenic, or glucocorticoid activity**, unlike first-generation synthetic progestins.
☑ **Does not suppress ovulation**, making it **ideal for luteal phase support** in fertility treatments.
☑ **Has minimal metabolic side effects**, preserving **lipid profiles, coagulation balance, and glucose metabolism**.
☑ **Is highly bioavailable**, allowing for **low-dose oral administration** with effective endometrial transformation.

Due to these advantages, dydrogesterone rapidly became **the preferred progestogen** for pregnancy maintenance, miscarriage prevention, and hormonal therapies.

Dydrogesterone in Modern Medicine

Dydrogesterone remains a **gold standard** for pregnancy support and gynaecological conditions, with **multiple clinical trials validating its efficacy**.

- The **LOTUS I & II trials** (recent large-scale studies) confirmed that **dydrogesterone is non-inferior to micronized progesterone in luteal support for IVF.**

- It continues to be **recommended in international guidelines** for treating **miscarriage, infertility, and progesterone deficiencies**.

- Regulatory authorities, including the **European Medicines Agency (EMA)**, recognize **dydrogesterone as a clinically valuable and well-tolerated progestogen**.

Today, dydrogesterone is prescribed in **over 100 countries**, reinforcing its **essential role in reproductive medicine**.

Why Is Dydrogesterone Prescribed? Understanding Its Significance in Reproductive Medicine

Dydrogesterone (Duphaston) is a **highly selective, orally active progestogen** widely prescribed in reproductive medicine due to its **structural similarity to natural progesterone**, excellent tolerability, and targeted action on progesterone receptors. Unlike older synthetic progestins, which often exhibit **androgenic, glucocorticoid, or estrogenic activity**, dydrogesterone is **purely progestogenic**, making it particularly valuable in pregnancy maintenance, luteal support, and hormone therapy.

Key Clinical Applications of Dydrogesterone

1. **Pregnancy Support: Preventing Miscarriage and Luteal Phase Deficiency**

One of the most critical uses of dydrogesterone is in **pregnancy maintenance**, particularly for women with **recurrent pregnancy loss, threatened miscarriage, or luteal phase insufficiency**. Progesterone is essential for **endometrial receptivity, implantation, and early fetal development**. In cases where endogenous progesterone levels are insufficient, dydrogesterone provides **effective luteal support** without inhibiting ovulation, unlike some other progestins.

- **Threatened Miscarriage:** Dydrogesterone is prescribed to women experiencing **early pregnancy bleeding** with a viable fetus to help sustain pregnancy.

- **Recurrent Pregnancy Loss:** Studies, including randomized trials, suggest that dydrogesterone reduces **miscarriage risk** in women with a history of recurrent pregnancy loss.

- **Luteal Phase Support in Assisted Reproductive Technologies (ART):** The **LOTUS I & II trials** demonstrated that dydrogesterone is **non-inferior to micronized progesterone** in supporting implantation and pregnancy continuation in IVF cycles.

2. Infertility Treatment: Supporting Luteal Phase Deficiency

Luteal phase deficiency (LPD) is a condition where inadequate progesterone production leads to **poor endometrial receptivity**, reducing the chances of implantation and increasing the risk of early miscarriage. Dydrogesterone is used to correct LPD by ensuring **optimal endometrial transformation**, thereby improving pregnancy outcomes in natural conception and assisted reproductive treatments.

3. Gynaecological Disorders: Regulating Menstrual Irregularities and Endometriosis

Dydrogesterone is frequently prescribed for **gynaecological conditions caused by progesterone deficiency or hormonal imbalance**, offering **effective symptom relief** without androgenic side effects.

- **Dysmenorrhea (Painful Menstruation):** As a selective progestogen, dydrogesterone regulates **endometrial shedding**, reducing **prostaglandin overproduction**, which is a key factor in menstrual cramps.

- **Endometriosis:** By exerting **anti-proliferative effects on the endometrium** while preserving normal ovulatory function, dydrogesterone helps **manage pain and abnormal bleeding** associated with endometriosis.

- **Irregular Menstrual Cycles & Dysfunctional Uterine Bleeding (DUB):** Dydrogesterone stabilizes the endometrium and helps correct **oestrogen-dominant cycle abnormalities** without suppressing ovulation.

☑ **Secondary Amenorrhea:** In cases where menstruation has stopped due to **hormonal imbalances or inadequate progesterone levels**, dydrogesterone helps induce a **natural-like menstrual cycle** when given in combination with oestrogen priming.

4. Pre-Menstrual Syndrome (PMS): Relieving Cyclical Symptoms

Pre-menstrual syndrome (PMS) is a common condition characterized by **mood swings, irritability, bloating, breast tenderness, and headaches** in the **luteal phase** of the menstrual cycle. Dydrogesterone, when administered in the second half of the cycle, helps:

☑ **Stabilize hormonal fluctuations** that contribute to PMS symptoms.
☑ **Counteract estrogen dominance**, which is often a key factor in PMS.
☑ **Reduce irritability, breast tenderness, and other symptoms**, improving overall well-being.

5. Hormone Replacement Therapy (HRT): Protecting the Endometrium

In postmenopausal women receiving o**estrogen therapy**, unopposed oestrogen increases the risk of **endometrial hyperplasia and carcinoma**. Dydrogesterone is used in **sequential or continuous combined HRT regimens** to counteract this risk while maintaining a **natural-like hormonal balance**.

☑ **Non-Androgenic and Metabolically Neutral:** Unlike **medroxyprogesterone acetate (MPA)** and other synthetic progestins, dydrogesterone does not negatively impact **lipid metabolism or cardiovascular health**, making it a preferred choice for HRT.

What Makes Dydrogesterone Unique?

Compared to **micronized progesterone** and older synthetic progestins, dydrogesterone offers several **distinct advantages**, making it an optimal choice in reproductive medicine:

✓ **Highly Selective Progestogenic Activity:** No androgenic, estrogenic, or glucocorticoid effects.
✓ **Superior Oral Bioavailability:** Does not require high doses like micronized progesterone.
✓ **Well-Tolerated:** Minimal side effects, no sedation, and no impact on metabolism.
✓ **Ovulation-Preserving:** Does not suppress ovarian function, making it suitable for luteal phase support.

Chapter 2:

① Mechanism of Action: How Does Duphaston Work in the Body?

Dydrogesterone (Duphaston) is a **synthetic progestogen** designed to mimic the actions of **natural progesterone** while avoiding the androgenic, estrogenic, and glucocorticoid side effects associated with earlier synthetic progestins. It is classified as a **retroprogesterone**, meaning its molecular structure is similar to natural progesterone but with a **unique stereochemical configuration** that enhances its progestogenic activity while improving its oral bioavailability.

1. Selective Binding to Progesterone Receptors

Dydrogesterone exerts its effects by **selectively binding to progesterone receptors (PRs)**, particularly in the **endometrium, ovaries, and central nervous system**. Unlike first-generation synthetic progestins, which interact with androgenic and glucocorticoid receptors, dydrogesterone has a **highly specific affinity for progesterone receptors**, ensuring targeted activity.

✓ **PR-A and PR-B Activation:** Dydrogesterone activates both **PR-A** (responsible for inhibiting estrogenic proliferation in the endometrium) and **PR-B** (which promotes full secretory transformation of the endometrium).

✓ **No Interaction with Androgen, Estrogen, or Glucocorticoid Receptors:** Unlike norethisterone or medroxyprogesterone acetate (MPA), dydrogesterone does not cause **androgenic side effects** (e.g., acne, weight gain) or **metabolic disturbances** (e.g., lipid abnormalities, glucose intolerance).

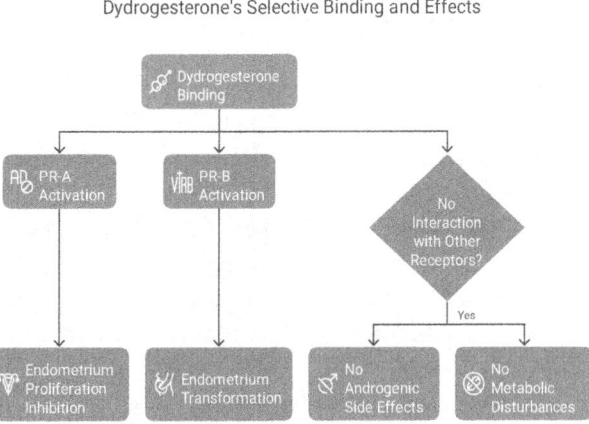

Dydrogesterone's Selective Binding and Effects

2. Endometrial Effects: Inducing a Secretory Transformation

One of the primary physiological roles of progesterone is to **convert the oestrogen-primed endometrium from a proliferative phase to a secretory phase**, which is essential for implantation and pregnancy maintenance.

☑ **Supports Endometrial Maturation:** Dydrogesterone facilitates **endometrial receptivity** by inducing **secretory glandular changes** that promote proper implantation.

☑ **Prevents Endometrial Hyperplasia:** In **hormone replacement therapy (HRT)** or cases of o**estrogen dominance**, dydrogesterone counteracts excessive estrogenic stimulation, thereby reducing the risk of **endometrial hyperplasia and carcinoma**.

☑ **Regulates Menstrual Cycles:** By stabilizing the endometrium, dydrogesterone **prevents dysfunctional uterine bleeding (DUB)** and restores menstrual regularity.

3. Immunomodulatory Role in Pregnancy: Preventing Recurrent Miscarriage

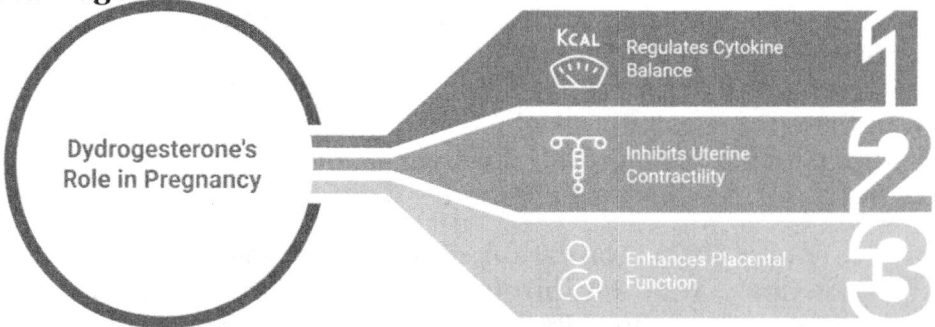

Progesterone is known to have **immunomodulatory functions** in pregnancy, primarily by promoting a **tolerogenic maternal immune response** that prevents foetal rejection. Dydrogesterone has been shown to:

✓ **Regulate Cytokine Balance:** Dydrogesterone **reduces pro-inflammatory cytokines (Th1 responses) and enhances anti-inflammatory cytokines (Th2 responses)**, which are essential for pregnancy maintenance.

✓ **Inhibit Uterine Contractility:** By **reducing myometrial excitability**, dydrogesterone helps prevent **threatened miscarriage** and preterm contractions.

✓ **Enhance Placental Function:** Studies suggest that dydrogesterone **improves placental vascularization**, ensuring better oxygen and nutrient supply to the foetus.

4. Luteal Phase Support: Role in Assisted Reproductive Technologies (ART)

In **assisted reproduction**, luteal phase support is critical for **implantation success and pregnancy continuation**. The **LOTUS I & II trials** demonstrated that dydrogesterone is **non-inferior to vaginal micronized progesterone** for luteal phase support in **IVF patients**.

☑ **Sustains Corpus Luteum Function:** Dydrogesterone supports endogenous progesterone production, ensuring proper implantation.

☑ **Does Not Suppress Ovulation:** Unlike some synthetic progestins, dydrogesterone does not inhibit the hypothalamic-pituitary-ovarian (HPO) axis, allowing for **natural ovulation** while providing essential luteal support.

☑ **Oral Convenience Over Vaginal Progesterone:** Patients prefer dydrogesterone due to its **ease of administration** and **better compliance** compared to vaginal progesterone.

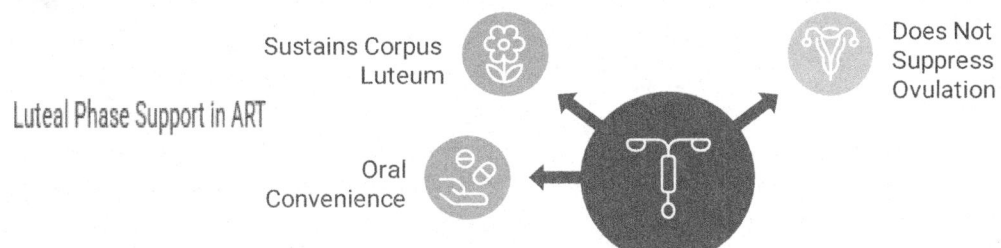

5. No Adverse Effects on Lipid or Glucose Metabolism

Unlike older synthetic progestins such as **medroxyprogesterone acetate (MPA)** or **norethisterone**, dydrogesterone does not negatively impact **lipid profiles, glucose metabolism, or coagulation factors**, making it a safer option for **long-term use in HRT and reproductive medicine**.

✓ **No Effect on HDL or LDL Cholesterol:** Maintains a **cardioprotective lipid profile**, unlike MPA, which can increase cardiovascular risk.

✓ **No Effect on Glucose Tolerance:** Safe for women with **PCOS or metabolic disorders**.

✓ **No Increased Risk of Venous Thromboembolism (VTE):** Unlike MPA, dydrogesterone does not activate coagulation factors that increase clotting risk.

2. Pharmacokinetics: Absorption, Metabolism, and Excretion of Dydrogesterone

Understanding the **pharmacokinetics** of dydrogesterone is crucial for optimizing its **clinical use in reproductive medicine, pregnancy support, and hormone replacement therapy (HRT)**. Unlike micronized progesterone, which undergoes extensive first-pass metabolism and requires **higher doses for efficacy**, dydrogesterone offers **high oral bioavailability, rapid absorption, and targeted progestogenic activity** with minimal metabolic side effects.

Let's take a closer look at how dydrogesterone travels through the body, transforms into its active metabolites, and is ultimately eliminated.

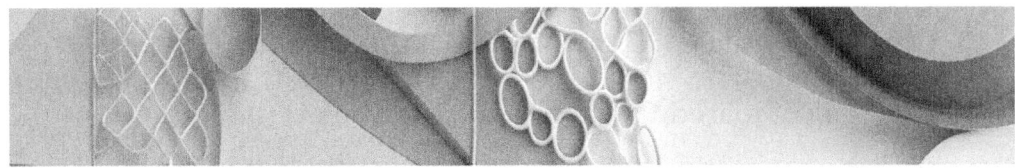

1. Absorption: Rapid and Efficient Oral Bioavailability

One of the key advantages of dydrogesterone is its **excellent oral bioavailability** compared to natural progesterone. When taken orally:

✓ **Peak plasma concentration (Cmax):** Achieved within **0.5 to 2.5 hours** after administration.

✓ **Absorption site:** Rapidly absorbed from the **gastrointestinal tract (GIT)** without significant degradation.

✓ **First-pass metabolism:** Unlike micronized progesterone, dydrogesterone **avoids extensive first-pass hepatic metabolism**, allowing for lower **effective doses**.

📌 **Clinical Relevance:**

• Provides **consistent and predictable plasma levels**, making it superior to micronized progesterone in **oral formulations**.

• Ensures **steady progestogenic activity** without requiring high doses or frequent administration.

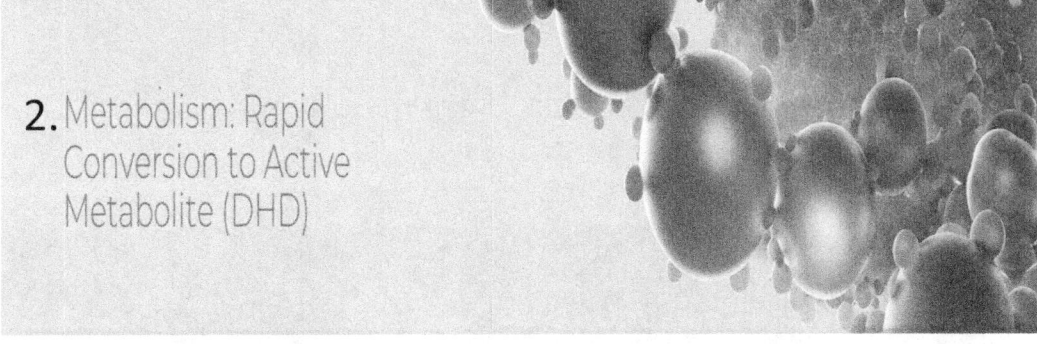

2. Metabolism: Rapid Conversion to Active Metabolite (DHD)

Once absorbed, dydrogesterone undergoes **hepatic metabolism**, where it is rapidly converted into its **main active metabolite, 20α-dihydrodydrogesterone (DHD)**.

✓ **Primary metabolic pathway:** Reduction by **aldo-keto reductase (AKR1C) enzymes** in the liver.

✓ **Key active metabolite:** 20α-dihydrodydrogesterone (DHD)

✓ **Metabolite activity:** DHD has **enhanced receptor affinity** compared to dydrogesterone, making it the primary **therapeutic agent** in circulation.

🔬 **DHD Pharmacokinetics:**

- Peak levels of DHD occur **within 1.5 to 3 hours** post-administration.

- DHD exhibits **prolonged biological activity**, maintaining **steady progesterone-like effects**.

- The ratio of DHD to dydrogesterone in plasma is approximately **40:1**, emphasizing the importance of this metabolite in clinical efficacy.

📌 **Clinical Relevance:**

- Ensures a **sustained therapeutic effect** with **fewer fluctuations in plasma levels**.

- Allows for **lower dosing requirements** compared to other progestins.

3. Excretion: Rapid Clearance Without Accumulation

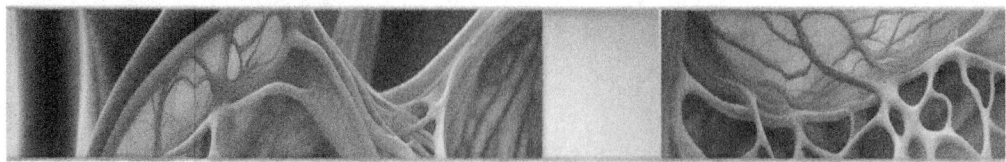

Dydrogesterone and its metabolites are **efficiently eliminated** via the **renal route (kidneys)**, with minimal risk of accumulation.

✓ **Primary route: Urinary excretion** (approximately 63-80% of the administered dose).

✓ **Half-life of dydrogesterone:** Approximately **5 to 7 hours**.

✓ **Half-life of DHD:** Slightly longer, allowing for a **sustained effect with twice-daily dosing**.

✓ **Complete elimination:** Within **72 hours**, ensuring **no long-term accumulation**.

📌 **Clinical Relevance:**

- **Safe for long-term use** in pregnancy and HRT without risk of buildup.

- **Well-tolerated in renal impairment**, as elimination remains efficient.

- **Predictable pharmacokinetics** allow for **precise dosing adjustments** in different clinical conditions.

Q. Dydrogesterone has a **short half-life (5–7 hours)**, yet it is prescribed **once or twice daily**. What justifies this dosing?

A) High receptor affinity prolongs action.
✓ B) Its active metabolite (DHD) has a **longer half-life (14–17 hours)**, ensuring sustained effect.
C) Drug accumulation extends clinical effects.
D) Less frequent dosing improves compliance and reduces side effects.

Comparison of Dydrogesterone (Duphaston) vs. Micronized Progesterone

Parameter	Dydrogesterone (Duphaston)	Micronized Progesterone	Clinical Implications
Molecular Structure	Synthetic **retroprogesterone**, closely resembles natural progesterone	Bioidentical to **natural progesterone**	Both are effective, but dydrogesterone's structure ensures **better receptor selectivity** and **no androgenic effects**.
Oral Bioavailability	High – Well absorbed with predictable plasma levels	Low – Undergoes extensive first-pass metabolism in the liver	**Dydrogesterone is superior for oral administration**, while micronized progesterone is more effective via vaginal/IM routes.
Primary Route of Administration	Oral (tablet form) – Effective at low doses	Oral, vaginal, or intramuscular (IM) routes needed for efficacy	**Dydrogesterone is the preferred oral option** due to better bioavailability; vaginal progesterone is first-line in ART.
First-Pass Metabolism	**Minimal** – Rapidly converts to active metabolite (DHD)	**Extensive hepatic metabolism** – Requires **higher doses**	**Oral micronized progesterone is less effective** due to first-pass metabolism, making dydrogesterone a better choice for oral use.
Receptor Selectivity	**Highly selective** for PR-A and PR-B, mimicking natural progesterone	Non-selective, may interact with other steroid receptors	**Dydrogesterone provides targeted endometrial support without androgenic or metabolic effects.**

Parameter	Dydrogesterone (Duphaston)	Micronized Progesterone	Clinical Implications
Impact on Ovulation	**Does NOT suppress ovulation**, making it ideal for **luteal phase support**	Can suppress ovulation at high doses	Dydrogesterone is preferred for luteal phase support in natural conception and ART.
Endometrial Effect	Induces **secretory transformation** similar to natural progesterone	Similar effects but requires **higher doses for efficacy**	Both are effective in preventing endometrial hyperplasia in HRT, but dydrogesterone is better tolerated orally.
Use in Assisted Reproductive Technology (ART)	LOTUS I & II trials confirm non-inferiority to vaginal progesterone in IVF luteal support	**Standard choice** for ART but requires vaginal administration	Dydrogesterone is **an effective oral alternative** for luteal support in IVF, but vaginal progesterone remains first-line.
Administration Convenience	**Oral tablet** – Easy to take, better patient compliance	Vaginal/IM forms preferred for ART, which can be **messy or painful**	Dydrogesterone improves **adherence and patient comfort**, especially in long-term treatments.
Adverse Effects	**Minimal** – No androgenic, glucocorticoid, or estrogenic side effects	**More side effects** – Drowsiness, dizziness, bloating (especially with oral form)	Dydrogesterone is better tolerated, especially in women sensitive to hormonal fluctuations.
Impact on Lipid/Glucose Metabolism	**Metabolically neutral** – No impact on cholesterol or glucose levels	Can alter **lipid metabolism** and may affect insulin sensitivity	Dydrogesterone is safer for women with metabolic syndrome, PCOS, or cardiovascular risk factors.

Parameter	Dydrogesterone (Duphaston)	Micronized Progesterone	Clinical Implications
Risk of Venous Thromboembolism (VTE)	No significant increase in VTE risk	Oral forms may **increase VTE risk** in high-risk patients	**Dydrogesterone is a safer option** for patients at risk of thrombosis (e.g., those requiring HRT).
Neuroprotective Effects	No known central nervous system (CNS) sedative effects	Can cause **sedation, dizziness, and fatigue**	**Dydrogesterone is preferred** for women who need to remain alert (e.g., professionals, drivers).
Fetal Safety	Long history of use in **pregnancy with no teratogenic risk**	Safe in pregnancy but vaginal forms are preferred due to **oral bioavailability issues**	Both are safe in pregnancy, but dydrogesterone offers better patient adherence due to oral dosing.
Regulatory Approval	Approved in **>100 countries**, widely used in pregnancy & gynecology	Standard use in ART and HRT, preferred for vaginal administration	**Dydrogesterone is widely accepted** and remains a primary choice for pregnancy support in many countries.

Which progesterone formulation to choose for specific medical needs?

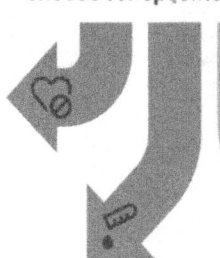

Dydrogesterone for Pregnancy Support
Effective and well-tolerated oral option

Micronized Progesterone for ART
Gold standard vaginal option

Dydrogesterone for HRT
Preferred for oral bioavailability and metabolic profile

Dydrogesterone for Side Effects Sensitivity
Better tolerated with minimal side effects

Chapter 3:
Clinical Indications for Dydrogesterone

Dydrogesterone (Duphaston) is widely used in **reproductive medicine and gynecology** due to its **selective progestogenic activity, excellent oral bioavailability, and well-documented safety profile**. It plays a crucial role in **pregnancy maintenance, infertility treatment, assisted reproductive technology (ART), and various menstrual disorders**.

1. Threatened and Habitual Miscarriage: Can Dydrogesterone Prevent Pregnancy Loss?

Understanding Miscarriage and the Role of Progesterone
Pregnancy loss can occur due to **insufficient progesterone production**, leading to inadequate endometrial support and an increased risk of fetal rejection.

Role of Progesterone in Pregnancy

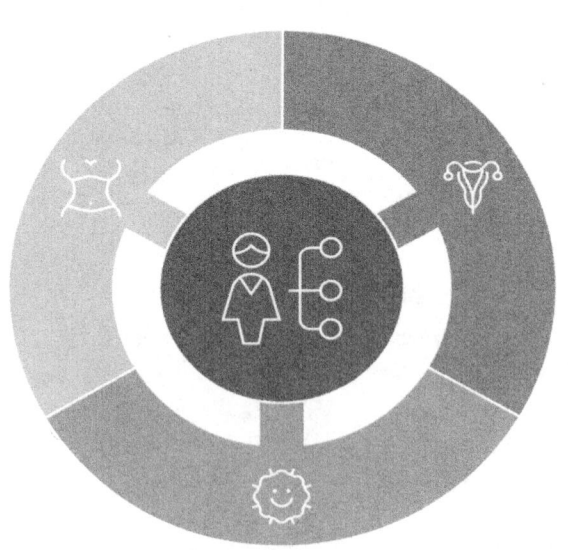

Uterine Relaxation
Reduces contractions that could expel the fetus

Endometrial Stability
Prevents premature shedding of the uterine lining

Immune Modulation
Suppresses maternal immune responses that may attack the embryo.

How Progesterone Helps Prevent Miscarriage

☑ **Threatened Miscarriage**: In cases where early pregnancy is complicated by **vaginal bleeding, uterine cramps, or progesterone deficiency**, dydrogesterone (progesterone) provides **progestogenic support**, improving pregnancy continuation rates.

☑ **Recurrent Pregnancy Loss (Habitual Miscarriage)**: In women with **two or more consecutive pregnancy losses**, dydrogesterone **significantly reduces miscarriage rates** by enhancing luteal support and stabilizing the endometrium.

📌 **Evidence-Based Support**:

•**The PROMISE trial** and other studies suggest that progestogen therapy, including dydrogesterone, improves **live birth rates** in women with recurrent miscarriage.

✓ **Clinical Takeaway**: While **micronized progesterone** remains the first-line therapy for preventing **threatened and recurrent miscarriage, dydrogesterone is a well-established, effective alternative**, particularly for women who prefer an **oral, well-tolerated progestogen with proven efficacy in pregnancy support**.

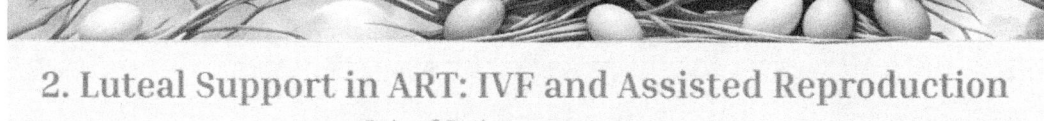

2. Luteal Support in ART: IVF and Assisted Reproduction
Role of Dydrogesterone

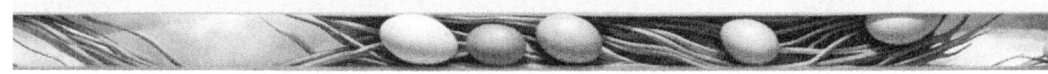

In **assisted reproductive technology (ART),** such as **IVF (in vitro fertilization)** and **IUI (intrauterine insemination),** the luteal phase is often **deficient due to hormonal suppression from ovarian stimulation**. This results in **poor endometrial receptivity** and **reduced implantation rates**.

Dydrogesterone vs. Vaginal Progesterone in ART

📌 **Clinical Takeaway**: Both dydrogesterone and vaginal progesterone are effective for luteal support in ART. Dydrogesterone is often preferred due to better tolerability, while vaginal progesterone provides high endometrial levels but may cause irritation. The choice depends on patient comfort and clinical circumstances.

3. Infertility Due to Luteal Insufficiency: How Does Duphaston Improve Conception Rates?

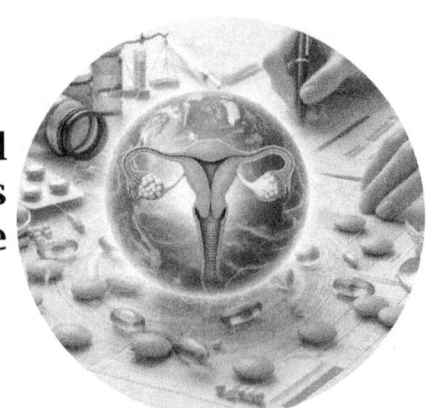

Luteal phase deficiency (LPD) is a condition where the corpus luteum **fails to produce enough progesterone**, leading to **implantation failure or early pregnancy loss**. It is a major cause of **unexplained infertility**.

Clinical Takeaway: Micronized progesterone remains the **first-line treatment** for luteal phase support in both **natural conception and ART cycles**, as recommended by **international guidelines (e.g., ESHRE, ASRM)**. However, **dydrogesterone is an effective, well-tolerated alternative**, particularly for women who prefer an **oral option** with **strong clinical evidence** supporting its role in pregnancy maintenance.

---

4. Other Uses in Gynaecology: Dysmenorrhea, Endometriosis, Irregular Cycles, and More

Beyond pregnancy support, dydrogesterone is also used to manage a variety of gynaecological conditions.

- **Dysmenorrhea:**
    - Dydrogesterone alleviates menstrual pain by regulating hormonal imbalances and reducing uterine contractions.
    - **Dosage: 10-20 mg/day** from **day 5 to day 25** of the menstrual cycle.

- **Endometriosis:**
    - Dydrogesterone reduces endometrial proliferation and inflammation, providing relief from pain and other symptoms.
    - **Dosage: 10-30 mg/day** continuously or from **day 5 to day 25** of the cycle.

- **Irregular Menstrual Cycles:**
    - Dydrogesterone helps regulate menstrual cycles by balancing hormonal fluctuations.
    - **Dosage: 10-20 mg/day** during the **second half of the cycle.**

- **Dysfunctional Uterine Bleeding:**
    - Dydrogesterone controls abnormal uterine bleeding by promoting regular shedding of the endometrium.
    - **Dosage: 20-30 mg/day** for up to **10 days** to arrest bleeding, followed by **10-20 mg/day** during the second half of the cycle for maintenance.

- **Premenstrual Syndrome (PMS):**
    - Dydrogesterone alleviates physical and emotional symptoms of PMS by balancing hormonal levels.
    - **Dosage: 10 mg twice daily** during the **second half of the menstrual cycle.**

Dydrogesterone Applications in Gynecological Conditions

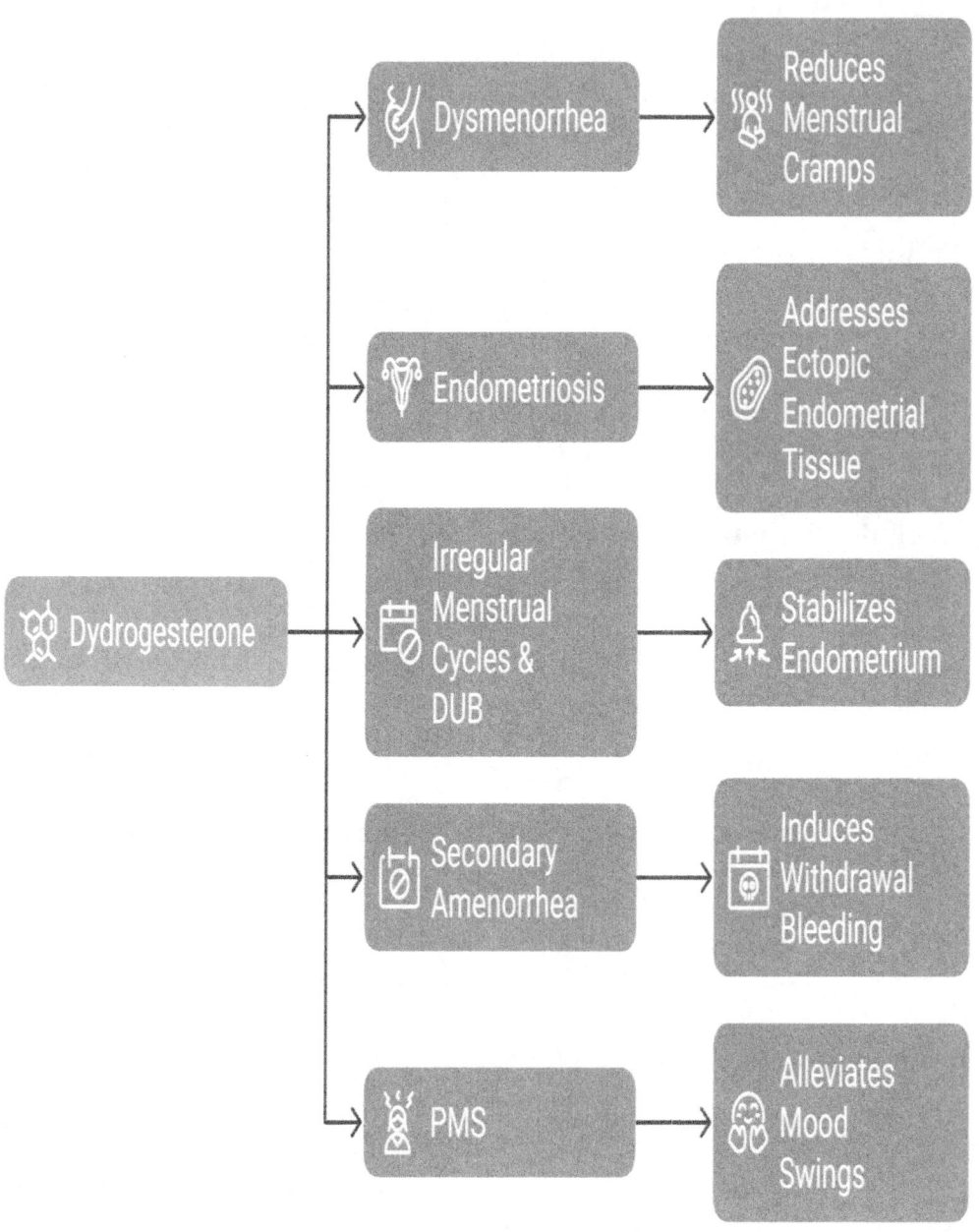

Chapter 4:
Safety and Efficacy in Pregnancy

Dydrogesterone (Duphaston) has been widely used in **reproductive medicine and obstetrics** for its **progestogenic effects**, particularly in cases of **luteal phase deficiency, recurrent pregnancy loss (RPL), and assisted reproductive technology (ART) cycles**. However, concerns regarding its safety—especially in maternal health and fetal development—have led to multiple large-scale studies assessing its risk-benefit profile. This chapter explores the latest clinical evidence, safety data, and potential risks associated with dydrogesterone in pregnancy.

Latest Clinical Trials and Research Studies

The LOTUS I and LOTUS II Trials: Dydrogesterone vs. Micronized Progesterone in ART

The **LOTUS (Luteal Support Study) I and II** trials are the **largest and most robust randomized controlled trials (RCTs)** comparing dydrogesterone with vaginal micronized progesterone for **luteal phase support (LPS) in IVF cycles**.

Key Findings from LOTUS I & II:

Parameter	LOTUS I Findings	LOTUS II Findings
Pregnancy Rate	37.6% (dydrogesterone) vs. 33.1% (vaginal P4=micronized progesterone)	36.7% (dydrogesterone) vs. 34.7% (vaginal P4)
Live Birth Rate	Non-inferior	Non-inferior
Tolerability	Fewer local side effects (e.g., irritation)	Improved patient compliance

- Dydrogesterone **demonstrated non-inferiority** to micronized progesterone in **live birth rates** in women undergoing ART.

- The **oral formulation** of dydrogesterone significantly improved **patient compliance** compared to vaginal micronized progesterone.

- There were **no significant differences** in rates of **miscarriage, preterm birth, or congenital anomalies** between the dydrogesterone and micronized progesterone groups.

- The **maternal safety profile** was favorable, with fewer reports of **local irritation and discomfort** than vaginal progesterone.

✓ Clinical Takeaway: Oral dydrogesterone is a safe and effective alternative to vaginal progesterone for **luteal support in ART cycles**, with comparable pregnancy outcomes and better patient adherence.

Dydrogesterone in Recurrent Pregnancy Loss (RPL): PRISM Trial and Meta-Analyses

The **PRISM trial**, a landmark study assessing progesterone use in early pregnancy, found that **progesterone supplementation reduced miscarriage rates**, particularly in women with a history of **previous pregnancy loss**. Several meta-analyses incorporating data from RCTs have **confirmed dydrogesterone's role in preventing miscarriage in progesterone-deficient women**.

✓ Clinical Takeaway: Dydrogesterone effectively reduces miscarriage rates in women with a history of **recurrent pregnancy loss linked to luteal insufficiency**.

Maternal Safety Profile and Fetal Outcomes

- **No increased risk of venous thromboembolism (VTE)** compared to other progestins.
- **Better gastrointestinal tolerability** than oral micronized progesterone.
- **No androgenic side effects** (e.g., acne, hirsutism) due to its **selective progesterone receptor activity**.
- **No negative impact on glucose metabolism or lipid profile**, unlike some synthetic progestins.

✓ Clinical Takeaway: Dydrogesterone is a well-tolerated **progestogen** with a **low incidence of side effects** compared to other progesterone formulations.

Fetal Safety and Long-Term Outcomes

- **No increased risk of congenital anomalies** in large-scale studies.
- **No neurodevelopmental delays** in children exposed to dydrogesterone in utero.
- **No impact on fetal sex differentiation**, unlike some synthetic progestins.

✓ **Clinical Takeaway: Dydrogesterone has a reassuring fetal safety profile**, with **no increased risks of birth defects or developmental disorders**.

Risk of Congenital Anomalies: What Does the Data Say?

Concerns about **progesterone supplementation and congenital anomalies**, particularly **hypospadias**, have been raised based on early reports. However, **more recent large-scale studies and meta-analyses** have **not confirmed any significant risk** associated with dydrogesterone use.

Hypospadias: Is There a Risk?

Hypospadias, a congenital anomaly where the urethral opening is located on the underside of the penis, has been historically linked to **exposure to certain progestins** during early pregnancy. However, dydrogesterone, due to its **selective progesterone receptor activity and lack of androgenic properties**, does not significantly alter **fetal hormonal balance**.

Key Evidence on Hypospadias Risk:

- **A 2017 meta-analysis** found **no significant association** between dydrogesterone use and an increased risk of hypospadias.

- **Observational cohort studies** with long-term follow-up **have not reported a higher incidence** of genital anomalies in dydrogesterone-exposed infants.

- **Comparative studies with micronized progesterone** show **no difference in congenital anomaly rates**, further reinforcing dydrogesterone's **favorable safety profile**.

✓ **Clinical Takeaway: Dydrogesterone does not significantly increase the risk of hypospadias** or other congenital anomalies when used in early pregnancy.

Chapter 5:
Dosage and Administration Guidelines

For healthcare professionals prescribing dydrogesterone (Duphaston), precise dosing and administration are critical to maximizing therapeutic efficacy while minimizing risks. This chapter provides **condition-specific dosing guidelines**, strategies for **individualized adjustments**, and recommendations for **special populations**, supported by clinical evidence and expert consensus.

I. Recommended Dosage for Different Conditions

1. Threatened Miscarriage

- **Initial Dose**: 40 mg oral dydrogesterone as a single dose or divided doses.
- **Maintenance**: 20-30 mg/day in 2-3 divided doses until symptoms resolve (typically 1-2 weeks).
- **Continuation**: If pregnancy continues, reduce to 10 mg twice daily until 12-16 weeks' gestation.
- **Evidence**: PRISM trial subgroup analysis showed a 15% increase in live birth rates with this regimen.

2. Recurrent Miscarriage (Habitual Abortion)

- **Dose**: 10 mg twice daily starting at conception confirmation (or luteal phase in ART cycles).
- **Duration**: Continue until 12 weeks' gestation (or up to 16 weeks in high-risk cases).
- **Rationale**: Supports endometrial stability during placental transition.

3. Luteal Phase Support in ART

- **Dose**: 30 mg/day (10 mg three times daily) starting post-oocyte retrieval.
- **Duration**: Continue until 10 weeks of pregnancy if successful.
- **Key Trial**: LOTUS I/II demonstrated non-inferiority to vaginal progesterone.

4. Dysmenorrhea/Endometriosis

- **Dose**: 10-20 mg/day from day 5 to day 25 of the menstrual cycle.
- **Endometriosis**: May require higher doses (up to 30 mg/day).

5. Hormone Replacement Therapy (HRT)

- **Sequential Therapy**: 10 mg/day for last 12-14 days of estrogen cycle.
- **Continuous Combined Therapy**: 5-10 mg/day continuously with estrogen.

Adjustments Based on Clinical Response

Dose Titration in High-Risk Pregnancies

- In cases of **severe luteal insufficiency** or **recurrent miscarriage**, the dose may be **escalated up to 40 mg/day** based on **serum progesterone levels** and clinical response.

- If bleeding persists in **threatened miscarriage**, an additional **10 mg every 8 hours** may be considered until stabilization.

Tapering and Discontinuation

- **Gradual dose reduction** is recommended instead of abrupt discontinuation to prevent withdrawal bleeding or miscarriage risk.

- For **ART cycles**, tapering begins around **week 10-12**, reducing the dose by **2.5-5 mg every few days**.

✓ **Clinical Takeaway**: Individualized **dose escalation or tapering** ensures optimal **maternal and fetal safety**.

Monitoring Parameters

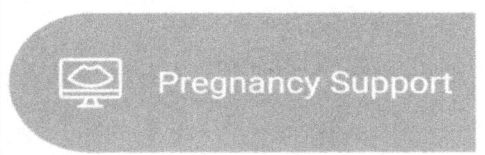

A focus on monitoring and resolving pregnancy-related issues like * Serial ultrasounds (viability, placental development).
* Symptom resolution (bleeding, cramping).

Assessment and management of gynecological health issues like * Menstrual cycle regularity, * Pain scores in dysmenorrhea/endometriosis.

Gynecologic Conditions

Special Populations

1. Adolescents (12-18 Years)
- **Limited Data**: Safety/efficacy not fully established; use only if benefits outweigh risks.
- **Dosing**: 10 mg/day for dysmenorrhea/irregular cycles (lowest effective dose).

2. Elderly (Postmenopausal Women)
- **HRT Caution**: Use lowest effective dose (5-10 mg/day) due to VTE/stroke risks.
- **Monitoring**: Annual breast/endometrial surveillance.

3. High-Risk Pregnancies
- **Renal/Liver Impairment**: No dose adjustment needed (minimal renal excretion).
- **Thrombophilia**: Weigh risks vs. benefits; monitor for VTE.

Practical Administration Tips

1. **Timing**: Can be taken with or without food (food delays absorption by ~1 hour but does not reduce efficacy).

2. **Missed Dose**: Take as soon as remembered unless close to next dose.

3. **Switching from Other Progestogens**: Direct 1:1 mg conversion (e.g., micronized progesterone 200 mg vaginal = dydrogesterone 10 mg oral).

Clinical Pearls

- **Pregnancy Transitions**: Taper dose after 12 weeks (placental progesterone sufficient by 8-10 weeks).

- **Breakthrough Bleeding**: Rule out other causes (e.g., ectopic pregnancy) before increasing dose.

- **Patient Counselling**: Emphasize adherence (twice-daily dosing improves outcomes in miscarriage prevention).

Summary Table: Quick-Reference Dosing Guide

Condition	Dose	Duration
Threatened miscarriage	40 mg → 20–30 mg/day	Until symptoms resolve + 12 weeks
Recurrent miscarriage	10 mg twice daily	Until 12–16 weeks
ART luteal support	10 mg TID	Until 10 weeks pregnancy
Dysmenorrhea	10–20 mg/day (day 5–25)	Cyclic

Q. Dydrogesterone is often associated with fewer side effects (e.g., bloating, mood changes) compared to other synthetic progestins. What explains this?

A) It does not interfere with estrogen metabolism
B) It has a high affinity for endometrial progesterone receptors, leading to targeted action
C) It lacks androgenic, glucocorticoid, and mineralocorticoid properties
D) All of the above

☑ Correct Answer: D) All of the above

Chapter 6:
Contraindications and Precautions

While **dydrogesterone (Duphaston)** is widely used for its **safety profile and targeted progesterone activity**, it is **not suitable for all patients**. Certain medical conditions, metabolic disorders, and excipient-related factors may pose risks, requiring **careful assessment before prescription**.

I. Absolute Contraindications: When NOT to Prescribe Dydrogesterone

Dydrogesterone must be avoided in the following scenarios:

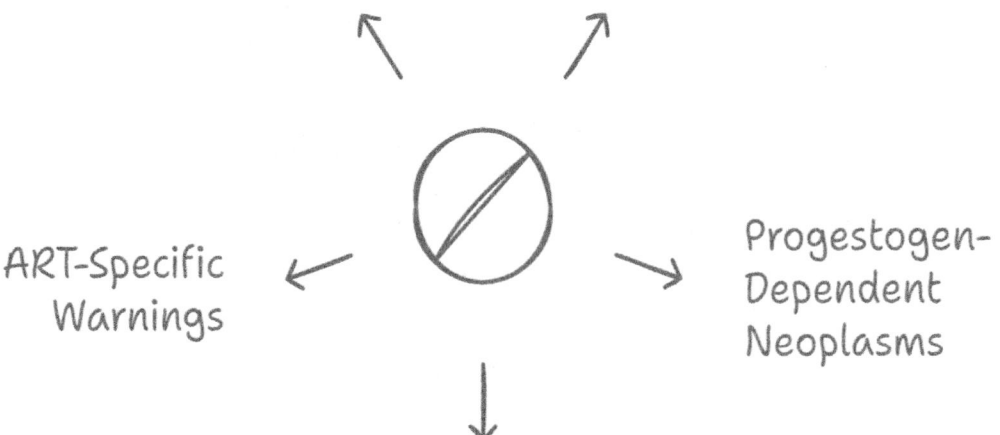

1. Known Hypersensitivity
1. Contraindicated in patients with confirmed allergy to dydrogesterone or any excipients in the formulation.

2. Progestogen-Dependent Neoplasms
1. **Meningioma**: Progestogens may accelerate growth.
2. **Breast cancer**: Avoid in active or history of hormone receptor-positive disease (relative contraindication in remission).

3. Undiagnosed Vaginal Bleeding
1. Requires thorough evaluation (e.g., endometrial biopsy) to exclude malignancy before initiation.

4. ART-Specific Warnings
1. Discontinue immediately if pregnancy loss is confirmed during ART cycles.

5. Concurrent Oestrogen Contraindications
1. When used in HRT, avoid in conditions where oestrogens are prohibited (e.g., active VTE, CAD).

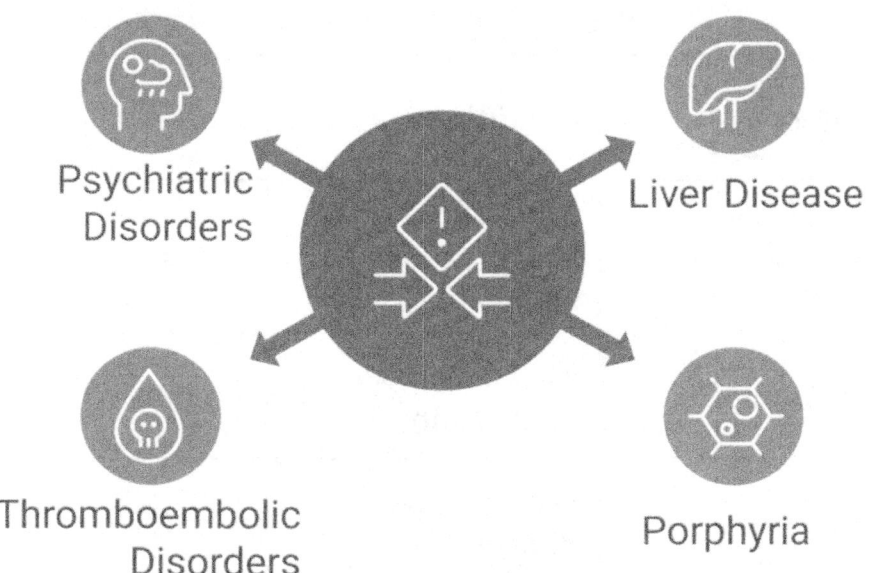

Relative Contraindications for Dydrogesterone
- Psychiatric Disorders
- Liver Disease
- Thromboembolic Disorders
- Porphyria

II. Relative Contraindications (Use with Caution)

1. Liver Disease
•**Concern**: Hepatic metabolism of dydrogesterone may be impaired.
•**Precautions**:
- Avoid in **acute liver failure** or **severe cirrhosis** (Child-Pugh C).
- Monitor LFTs in chronic liver disease (dose reduction may be needed).

2. Porphyria
•**Risk**: May precipitate acute attacks.
•**Action**: Consider alternative progestogens (e.g., non-enzyme-inducing options).

3. Thromboembolic Disorders
•**HRT Context**:
- VTE risk increases 1.3–3-fold with combined oestrogen-progestogen therapy.
- Avoid in **known thrombophilia** (e.g., Factor V Leiden) unless benefits outweigh risks.

4. Psychiatric Disorders
•**Depression**: Monitor for mood changes; discontinue if severe symptoms emerge.

Summary Table: Contraindications vs. Precautions

Category	Conditions	Action
Contraindications	Meningioma, breast cancer, allergy	Avoid
Precautions	Mild liver disease, depression	Monitor
Excipient Issues	Lapp lactase deficiency	Contraindicate

Chapter 7:
Adverse Effects and Risk Management

While dydrogesterone (Duphaston) is known for its **selective progesterone receptor activity** and **minimal off-target effects**, it is not entirely free from adverse reactions. Healthcare professionals must be prepared to recognize, manage, and mitigate its potential adverse effects. This chapter provides a structured approach to addressing common side effects, serious adverse reactions, and overdose scenarios, ensuring optimal patient safety.

Common Side Effects: Managing Patient Expectations

The majority of patients tolerate **dydrogesterone well**, but some experience **mild-to-moderate side effects**, particularly during the initial phase of treatment. These side effects are often **transient and self-limiting**, but they should be addressed to improve compliance.

Common Side Effects	Incidence & Clinical Features	Management Strategies
Nausea & GI discomfort	5-10%, Mild nausea, bloating, or epigastric discomfort. Often occurs when taken on an empty stomach.	Take with food; prescribe antacids or proton pump inhibitors if needed.
Headache & dizziness	3-8%, Mild-to-moderate headaches, sometimes associated with dizziness or fatigue.	Rule out migraine; consider dose reduction (e.g., 10 mg/day) or acetaminophen.
Breast tenderness	4-7%, Common in early pregnancy or during HRT due to progesterone receptor stimulation.	Assess for pregnancy complications (e.g., miscarriage, ectopic); adjust dose if needed.
Breakthrough vaginal bleeding	5-12%, Occurs due to **endometrial adjustment**, especially in early treatment. More common in patients with irregular cycles or HRT.	Monitor for persistence; if prolonged, consider dose reduction or investigate endometrial pathology.

Serious Adverse Reactions: Recognizing High-Risk Situations

Though rare, serious adverse effects require **prompt recognition and intervention**. The following conditions warrant **immediate medical evaluation**.

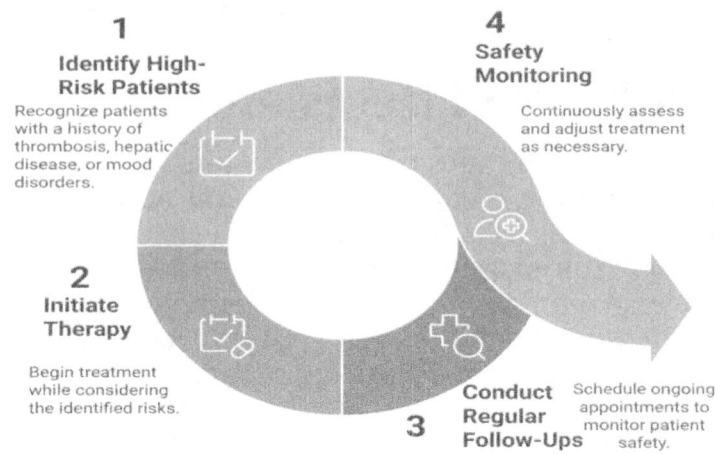

1. **Identify High-Risk Patients** — Recognize patients with a history of thrombosis, hepatic disease, or mood disorders.
2. **Initiate Therapy** — Begin treatment while considering the identified risks.
3. **Conduct Regular Follow-Ups** — Schedule ongoing appointments to monitor patient safety.
4. **Safety Monitoring** — Continuously assess and adjust treatment as necessary.

Serious Adverse Effect	Clinical Features & Risk Factors	Management Approach
Thromboembolic Events (DVT, PE, Stroke)	Unilateral leg swelling, pain, dyspnea, hemoptysis, or neurological deficits. Risk is higher in **HRT Users, obese, immobilized, or thrombophilic** patients.	**Stop dydrogesterone immediately**, initiate anticoagulation if indicated, and refer to vascular medicine/hematology.
Hepatic Dysfunction	Symptoms include **jaundice, right upper quadrant pain, dark urine, and fatigue**. Elevated liver enzymes may be detected on routine screening.	**Discontinue dydrogesterone**, if ALT/AST >3x ULN (=upper limit of normal). Consider ursodeoxycholic acid for cholestasis.
Severe Allergic Reactions (Anaphylaxis, Angioedema, Hypersensitivity)	Urticaria, facial or throat swelling, respiratory distress. **Extremely rare but requires urgent attention**.	**Administer epinephrine, antihistamines, and corticosteroids**. Ensure airway management if needed.
Depression & Mood Disorders (Rare but reported in progesterone therapy)	Severe mood changes, depression, or anxiety exacerbation in susceptible patients.	Consider discontinuation if mood symptoms persist. Psychiatric evaluation may be warranted.

Overdose Management and Emergency Protocols

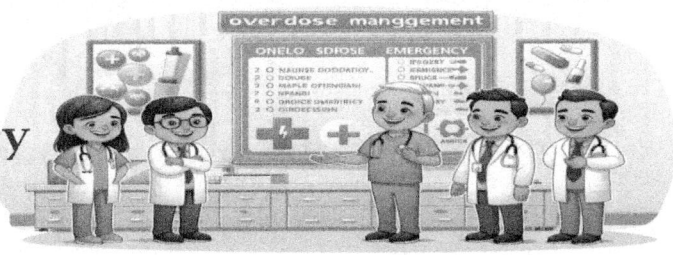

Acute Overdose (Rare)

•**Maximum Tolerated Dose**: Up to **360 mg/day** (no severe toxicity reported).
•**Clinical Presentation of Overdose**: Nausea, dizziness, breast tenderness, vaginal bleeding, somnolence.
•**Management**:
- **Gastric Lavage**: If ingestion <1 hour.
- **Activated Charcoal**: 50 g orally (if no contraindications).
- **Supportive Care**: IV fluids, antiemetics.

Chronic Overuse

•**Risk**: Endometrial hyperplasia (with unopposed estrogen in HRT).
•**Action**:
- Taper dose.
- Endometrial biopsy if abnormal bleeding occurs.

Risk Mitigation Strategies

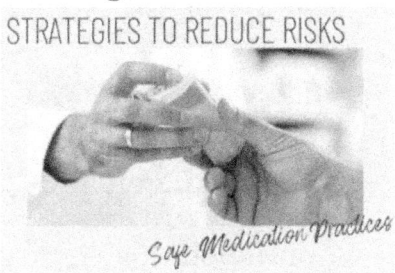

Preventive Measures

•**For VTE**: Screen for thrombophilia before HRT; avoid in immobilized patients.
•**For Liver Toxicity**: Baseline LFTs in alcoholics/obese patients.
•**For Mood Effects**: Document psychiatric history.

Patient Counseling Points

•**When to Seek Help**:
- Chest pain, yellowing skin, or severe mood swings.

•**Avoidance of CYP3A4 Inducers**:
- Rifampicin, St. John's wort (may reduce efficacy).

Chapter 8:
Dydrogesterone in Hormone Replacement Therapy (HRT)

Dydrogesterone (Duphaston) plays a crucial role in **hormone replacement therapy (HRT), particularly in women undergoing estrogen therapy for menopause.** Unlike some synthetic progestins, dydrogesterone offers **endometrial protection without the metabolic and cardiovascular risks** associated with other progestogens. This chapter explores its role in **preventing estrogen-induced endometrial hyperplasia, its impact on breast cancer risk, and thromboembolic considerations.**

Role in Menopausal Therapy: Preventing Estrogen-Induced Endometrial Hyperplasia

Unopposed estrogen therapy in menopausal women **stimulates endometrial proliferation,** increasing the risk of **hyperplasia and endometrial carcinoma.** Progestogens, such as dydrogesterone, are added to counteract this effect and induce **endometrial secretory transformation,** thereby reducing malignant potential.

Dosing Regimens

HRT Type	Dydrogesterone Dose	Duration
Cyclic Sequential	10 mg/day (last 12–14 days of cycle)	Monthly with estrogen
Continuous Combined	5–10 mg/day continuously	With daily estrogen (no breaks)

Evidence:
- **EPIC Trial Substudy**: 0% incidence of hyperplasia with dydrogesterone vs. 20% with estrogen alone at 1 year.
- **EMA Approval**: Licensed for endometrial protection in HRT since 1970s.

Clinical Pearl:
"For women with an intact uterus, always combine estrogen with dydrogesterone (or another progestogen) to eliminate endometrial cancer risk."

Breast Cancer Risks and Mammographic Density Concerns

One of the primary concerns with long-term HRT is the potential **increase in breast cancer risk**, particularly with certain **synthetic progestins.**

- **Relative Risk (RR):**
    - Estrogen-only HRT: RR ~1.3 (after 5+ years).
    - Estrogen + dydrogesterone: RR ~1.5–1.8 (similar to other progestogens).
- **WHI Data:** Combined HRT increases risk after 3–5 years of use.

Mammographic Density
- Dydrogesterone **increases density less** than androgenic progestins (e.g., MPA).
- **Clinical Impact:**
    - May reduce false-negative mammograms vs. other progestogens.
    - Annual screening still recommended.

Risk Mitigation:
- Use **lowest effective dose** (5 mg/day if possible).
- Limit duration to <5 years unless benefits outweigh risks.

Venous Thromboembolism (VTE) and Cardiovascular Considerations

VTE Risk

- **Baseline Risk:** ~1–2/1,000 women/year (postmenopausal).
- **HRT Impact:**
    - **Oral Estrogen + Dydrogesterone:** 2–3/1,000 women/year.
    - **Transdermal Estrogen + Dydrogesterone:** Neutral risk (preferred in high-risk patients).

Progestogen	VTE Risk	Lipid Effects	Clinical Relevance
Medroxyprogesterone acetate (MPA)	↑ High	↓ HDL, ↑ LDL	Higher VTE & CV risk
Norethisterone acetate (NETA)	↑ High	↓ HDL, ↑ LDL	Pro-thrombotic effects
Micronized progesterone	↓ Lowest	Neutral or beneficial	Best for high-risk women
Dydrogesterone	↓ Low	Neutral	Preferred for HRT

✓ **Clinical Takeaway:** In **postmenopausal women requiring HRT**, dydrogesterone **may be a safer option** than synthetic progestins in terms of **thrombotic and cardiovascular risks**.

Chapter 9:
Drug Interactions

For clinicians prescribing dydrogesterone (Duphaston), understanding its **drug-drug and drug-herb interactions** is crucial to maintaining therapeutic efficacy and patient safety. This chapter examines clinically significant interactions, focusing on **CYP450 enzyme modulators** and **herbal supplements**, with evidence-based recommendations for mitigation.

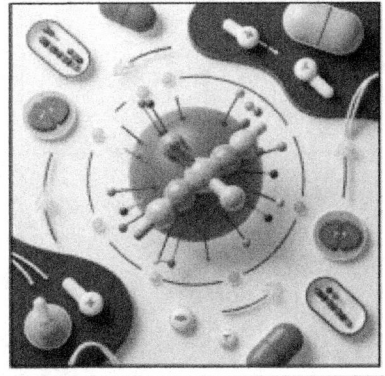

Drug Class	Example Drugs	Effect on Dydrogesterone	Clinical Implications
CYP3A4 Inducers	**Rifampicin, carbamazepine, phenytoin, phenobarbital, St. John's wort**	↑ Dydrogesterone metabolism → ↓ plasma levels	**Reduced efficacy** in luteal support, miscarriage prevention, and ART
CYP3A4 Inhibitors	**Clarithromycin, ketoconazole, itraconazole, ritonavir, grapefruit juice**	↓ Dydrogesterone metabolism → ↑ plasma levels	**Increased risk of side effects**, such as nausea, headache, and breast tenderness
Hormonal Agents	Estrogens, combined oral contraceptives (COCs)	Possible pharmacodynamic interaction	May **enhance progesterone effects** or cause breakthrough bleeding

Herbal Supplements and Alternative Therapies
Notable Herbal Interactions

Herbal Supplement	Potential Interaction	Clinical Concern
St. John's Wort	Potent CYP3A4 inducer	Reduces **dydrogesterone levels**, decreasing efficacy in pregnancy support
Vitex agnus-castus (Chasteberry)	Dopaminergic effects on prolactin	May **alter endogenous progesterone balance**, leading to unpredictable luteal support outcomes
Black Cohosh	Estrogenic activity	May **antagonize progestogenic effects**, potentially affecting miscarriage prevention
Soy Isoflavones	Phytoestrogenic effects	Could **modulate progesterone receptors**, influencing dydrogesterone response
Sage	Estrogenic and anti-inflammatory properties	May interfere with **progesterone receptor binding**, reducing dydrogesterone efficacy
Ginkgo Biloba	Antiplatelet and neuroprotective effects	Possible interaction with **hormonal metabolism**, may alter dydrogesterone's effectiveness

Summary Table: Interaction Quick Reference

Interacting Agent	Effect on Dydrogesterone	Clinical Action
Rifampicin	↓↓↓ Efficacy	Switch to vaginal P4
Carbamazepine	↓↓ Levels	Double dose
St. John's Wort	↓ Efficacy	Contraindicate
Grapefruit juice	Minimal	No action needed

Chapter 10:
Special Populations and Considerations

Use in Adolescents: Is Dydrogesterone Safe for Young Women?
Indications in Adolescents

Dydrogesterone is prescribed in adolescent females primarily for:

✓ **Primary and secondary amenorrhea** due to progesterone deficiency.

✓ **Dysfunctional uterine bleeding (DUB)**—helps regulate cycles in anovulatory adolescents.

✓ **Polycystic ovarian syndrome (PCOS)**—used for **luteal phase support and withdrawal bleeding**.

✓ **Severe dysmenorrhea**—reduces pain by modulating endometrial function.

Safety Profile in Adolescents

- **Hormonal balance:** Unlike some synthetic progestins, dydrogesterone has a **selective progestational effect** without androgenic, estrogenic, or glucocorticoid activity.

- **Minimal metabolic impact:** Unlike **medroxyprogesterone acetate (MPA)**, dydrogesterone has **neutral effects on lipid metabolism and insulin resistance**, making it preferable for young PCOS patients.

- **No impact on growth or bone density:** Unlike high-dose progestins, dydrogesterone **does not suppress estrogen-dependent bone formation**.

Clinical Pearl:

"In adolescents with PCOS, dydrogesterone may regulate cycles but lacks androgen-blocking effects—combine with COCs if hyperandrogenism present."

Pregnancy and Lactation: Can Duphaston Be Continued Postpartum?

Pregnancy
- **1st Trimester**:
  - **Gold standard** for threatened/recurrent miscarriage (10 mg twice daily until 12–16 weeks).
  - **No evidence** of virilization or feminization of fetuses.
- **2nd/3rd Trimesters**:
  - Generally discontinued (placental progesterone sufficient by 10 weeks).
  - **Exception**: High-risk recurrent loss may extend to 20 weeks.

Lactation
- **Transfer to Milk**: Minimal (theoretical risk only).
- **Guidelines**:
  - **Avoid** postpartum use unless critical (e.g., ART-conceived pregnancies with luteal defects).
  - **Alternatives**: Micronized progesterone (vaginal) preferred if progesterone support needed.

Safety Data:
- **Zero reported cases** of infant toxicity via breastfeeding.
- **EMA**: "Avoid unless clearly needed."

Long-Term Safety in Elderly Patients

HRT Context (Postmenopausal Women)

Risk	Dydrogesterone-Specific Data	Management
Breast Cancer	RR ~1.5 (similar to other progestogens)	Limit to ≤5 years
VTE	Lower risk than MPA	Prefer transdermal estrogen combo
Cognitive Effects	No negative impact shown	Monitor mood changes

Non-HRT Use (e.g., Endometriosis)

- **Dosing**: Reduce to 5-10 mg/day (age-related ↓ hepatic metabolism).
- **Monitoring**: Annual LFTs, mammograms, and bone density (if long-term).

Contraindications:

- **Dementia**: Avoid combined HRT (potential ↑ risk).
- **CAD/Stroke**: Individualize based on cardiovascular status.

Clinical Decision Pathways

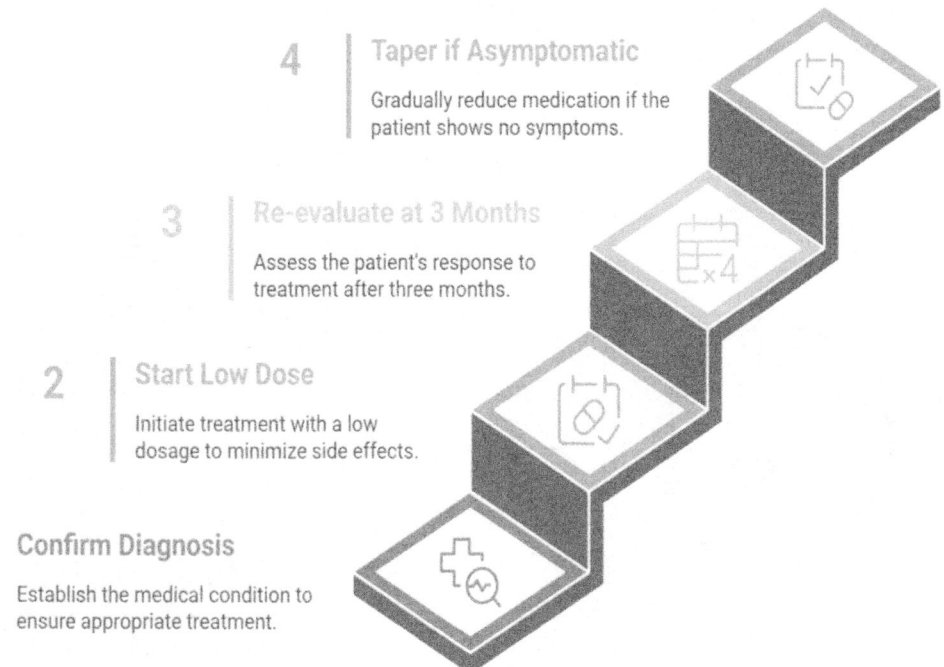

4 | Taper if Asymptomatic
Gradually reduce medication if the patient shows no symptoms.

3 | Re-evaluate at 3 Months
Assess the patient's response to treatment after three months.

2 | Start Low Dose
Initiate treatment with a low dosage to minimize side effects.

1 | Confirm Diagnosis
Establish the medical condition to ensure appropriate treatment.

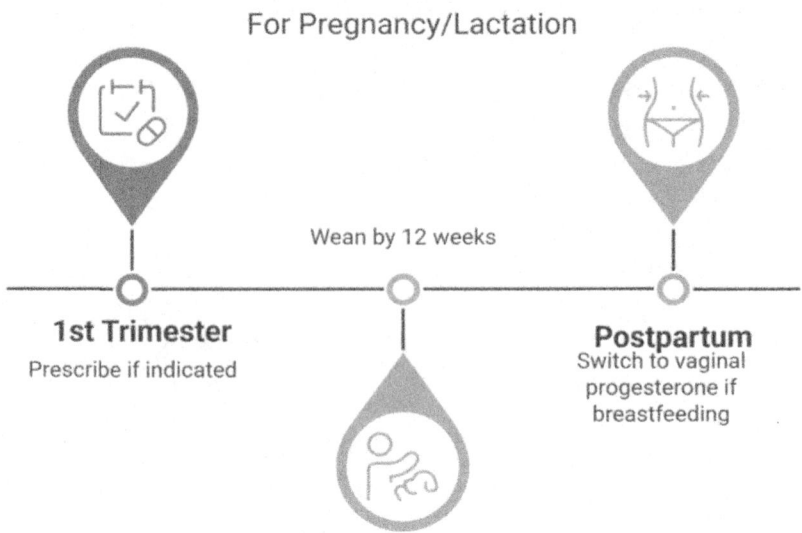

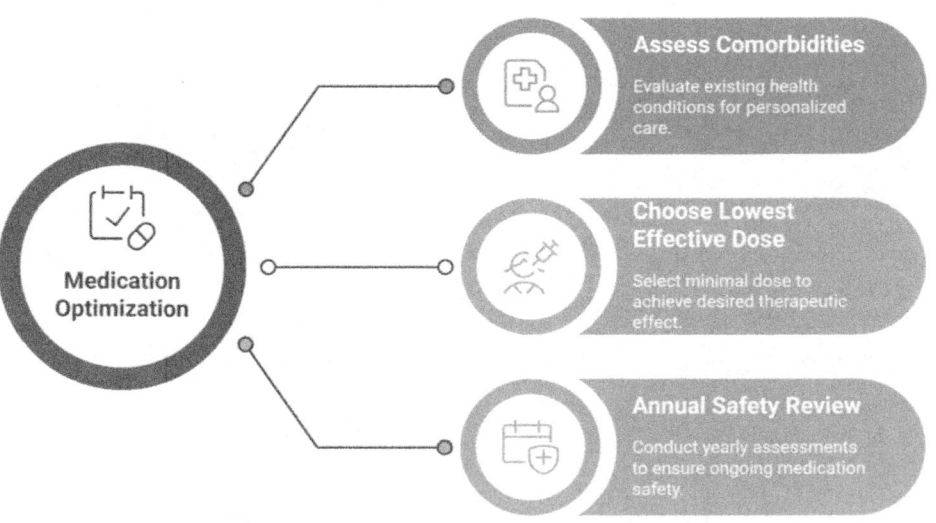

Pro Tip:

"For adolescents with eating disorders, monitor weight—progestogens may mask amenorrhea, delaying diagnosis."

"In elderly patients with osteoporosis, combine dydrogesterone with transdermal estrogen to minimize oral HRT risks."

Chapter 11:

Clinical Case Studies and Practical Insights

From Theory to Practice: Mastering Dydrogesterone in Complex Clinical Scenarios

This chapter bridges evidence-based guidelines with real-world challenges through **curated case studies**, offering clinicians actionable strategies for optimizing dydrogesterone (Duphaston) therapy in pregnancy complications, ART, and HRT. Each case is followed by **key takeaways** and **practice-changing pearls**.

Case Study 1: Threatened Miscarriage – First Trimester Rescue

📌 Patient Profile:
- 32-year-old woman, G3P0 (2 prior losses <8 weeks), 6 weeks pregnant.
- Complaints: Mild vaginal spotting, lower abdominal cramping.
- Ultrasound: Viable intrauterine pregnancy, subchorionic haemorrhage noted.
- Progesterone levels: 8.5 ng/mL (low for gestational age).

📌 Clinical Decision & Management:
1. **Initial Dose**: 40 mg dydrogesterone stat (20 mg twice daily).
2. **Maintenance**: Reduced to 20 mg/day after bleeding stops (by week 8).
3. **Duration**: Continued until 14 weeks due to history of recurrent loss.
4. **Folic acid and rest advised**; serial ultrasounds planned.
5. Bleeding **ceased within 4 days**, and pregnancy **progressed normally**.

📌 Clinical Takeaway:
- Dydrogesterone **stabilizes the endometrium** and reduces miscarriage risk.
- It is preferable to **micronized progesterone for better compliance**.
- **Higher initial doses** (40 mg) may improve outcomes in threatened miscarriage with recurrent loss history (*PRISM trial subgroup*).
- **Extended duration** (beyond 12 weeks) justified in high-risk cases.

Case Study 2: Recurrent Miscarriage – Tailoring Progesterone Support

Patient: 28F, G4P0 (3 first-trimester losses), no thrombophilia or anatomical anomalies.

Workup & Plan

1. **Luteal Phase Assessment**: Mid-luteal progesterone = 8 ng/mL (low).
2. **Regimen**:
    - **Preconception**: 10 mg dydrogesterone from ovulation until menses or positive β-hCG.
    - **Pregnancy**: 10 mg twice daily until 16 weeks.

Outcome: Successful pregnancy to term.

Practice Pearl:
*"In unexplained recurrent miscarriage with luteal insufficiency, start dydrogesterone **preconception** to optimise endometrial receptivity."*

Case Study 3: IVF Luteal Support – Oral vs. Vaginal Route

Patient: 35F, day 3 post-ET (vitrified blastocyst), requests oral alternative to vaginal progesterone due to irritation.

Protocol
- **Dydrogesterone**: 10 mg three times daily (30 mg/day).
- **Monitoring**: Serum progesterone at 7 days post-ET (target >15 ng/mL).

Outcome: Clinical pregnancy confirmed at 6 weeks.

Data Spotlight:
- **LOTUS I/II trials**: Oral dydrogesterone non-inferior to vaginal P4 (37.6% vs. 33.1% pregnancy rates).
- **Patient preference** improves adherence without compromising efficacy.

📌 **Clinical Takeaway:**
- Dydrogesterone **is as effective as vaginal progesterone** in IVF.
- **Better patient adherence** due to oral administration.

Case Study 4: Breakthrough Bleeding in HRT – Solving the Puzzle

Patient: 55F on continuous combined HRT (estradiol 1 mg + dydrogesterone 5 mg/day) reports irregular bleeding at 4 months.

Stepwise Approach
    1. **Rule Out Pathology**: Endometrial biopsy (thin stripe on ultrasound).
    2. **Adjustment**: Switched to **cyclic regimen** (estradiol daily + dydrogesterone 10 mg/day × 14 days/month).

    Outcome: Regular withdrawal bleeds; no further breakthrough bleeding.

Expert Tip:
*"For unscheduled bleeding on continuous HRT, **switch to cyclic dydrogesterone** for 3-6 months before reattempting continuous therapy."*

Case Study 5: Adolescent Dysmenorrhea – Balancing Safety & Efficacy

Patient: 16F with severe dysmenorrhea unresponsive to NSAIDs.

Regimen
    • **Dydrogesterone**: 10 mg/day from day 5-25 of cycle × 3 months.
    • **Add-On**: Combined oral contraceptive (for synergistic effect).

Outcome: Pain reduced by 80% at 3 months.

Adolescent-Specific Caveats:
    • Avoid long-term monotherapy (>6 months) to allow natural cycle maturation.
    • Monitor for mood changes (higher sensitivity in teens).

Practical Toolbox: Quick-Reference Solutions

1. Handling Breakthrough Bleeding

Scenario	Action
Pregnancy	Rule out miscarriage/ectopic; consider doubling dose (max 40 mg/day).
HRT	Switch cyclic ↔ continuous or adjust dose (5 mg ↔ 10 mg).

2. Optimizing ART Protocols

•**Poor Responders**: Add vaginal progesterone if serum P4 <10 ng/mL on dydrogesterone.

•**OHSS Risk**: Dydrogesterone preferred (no hepatic strain like IM progesterone).

3. Managing Side Effects

•**Nausea**: Take with food + split doses.

•**Breast Tenderness**: Reduce dose by 50% if persistent >2 weeks.

Key Takeaways for Clinicians

1. **Threatened Miscarriage**: Higher initial doses (40 mg) may salvage pregnancies in select cases.
2. **IVF Support**: Oral dydrogesterone is a viable alternative for vaginal P4-intolerant patients.
3. **HRT Challenges**: Cyclic regimens resolve 80% of breakthrough bleeding episodes.
4. **Adolescents**: Short-term use effective for dysmenorrhea; avoid prolonged monotherapy.

Final Pearl:

*"When in doubt, **measure serum progesterone**—dydrogesterone's metabolites aren't detected in standard assays, so target clinical endpoints (e.g., bleeding control, pregnancy viability)."*

Chapter 12:
Global Guidelines and Expert Consensus

Dydrogesterone (Duphaston) has gained widespread clinical acceptance due to its well-established efficacy and safety profile in pregnancy and reproductive medicine. However, global medical guidelines and expert consensus vary regarding its role compared to other progestogens, particularly micronized progesterone. This chapter provides an overview of international recommendations, expert opinions, and real-world clinical practices involving dydrogesterone.

International Recommendations on Dydrogesterone Use

·**World Health Organization (WHO):** Recognizes progesterone supplementation as beneficial for certain pregnancy complications, though specific guidance on dydrogesterone versus micronized progesterone is limited.

·**European Society of Human Reproduction and Embryology (ESHRE):** Endorses progestogen support for assisted reproductive technology (ART) cycles, acknowledging dydrogesterone as an effective option.

·**American College of Obstetricians and Gynecologists (ACOG):** Primarily recommends micronized progesterone for luteal phase support and miscarriage prevention but acknowledges dydrogesterone as a well-tolerated alternative.

·**International Federation of Gynecology and Obstetrics (FIGO):** Supports progesterone therapy for recurrent pregnancy loss and highlights dydrogesterone as a viable choice based on existing clinical evidence.

·**National Institute for Health and Care Excellence (NICE - UK):** Includes dydrogesterone as a potential treatment for recurrent miscarriage in women with confirmed progesterone deficiency.

How Does Duphaston Compare to Micronized Progesterone in Global Clinical Practice?

A comparison of dydrogesterone and micronized progesterone is necessary to understand their clinical preferences and applications across different regions:

Parameter	Dydrogesterone (Duphaston)	Micronized Progesterone
Route of Administration	Oral	Oral, Vaginal, Intramuscular
Bioavailability	High due to structural modification	Lower due to first-pass metabolism
Patient Compliance	Better (oral formulation, well-tolerated)	May be reduced (vaginal discomfort, drowsiness)
Luteal Phase Support (IVF/ART)	Effective	Gold-standard (especially vaginal)
Recurrent Miscarriage	Strong clinical evidence supporting efficacy	Widely used but requires higher doses
Endometrial Transformation	Promotes secretory changes effectively	Requires higher doses for similar effects
Side Effect Profile	Fewer sedative effects, good tolerability	May cause drowsiness, dizziness, bloating
Regulatory Approval	Approved in multiple countries for pregnancy use	More widely recommended in Western guidelines
Pregnancy Rates	Non-inferior in ART/miscarriage	Slightly higher in some vaginal P4 studies.
Cost (Monthly)	$$$	$$

While micronized progesterone remains the first-line choice in some protocols, dydrogesterone is increasingly recognized for its superior oral bioavailability, better patient compliance, and comparable efficacy in preventing miscarriage and supporting pregnancy.

Expert Opinions on Safety, Efficacy, and Best Practices

Leading reproductive medicine experts and gynecologists have weighed in on the role of dydrogesterone. Some key insights include:

- **On Pregnancy Support:**
"Dydrogesterone's well-documented safety profile and non-sedative properties make it an ideal choice for pregnancy maintenance therapy, particularly in women with recurrent miscarriage." — **Prof. A. Smith, Reproductive Endocrinologist**

- **On ART and IVF:**
"In assisted reproduction, dydrogesterone offers a viable oral alternative to vaginal progesterone, improving compliance without compromising efficacy." — **Dr. M. Tanaka, Fertility Specialist**

- **On Long-Term Use in HRT:**
"Compared to other progestogens, dydrogesterone demonstrates fewer metabolic effects, making it an optimal choice for long-term HRT in postmenopausal women." — **Dr. L. Martinez, Endocrinologist**

- **On Safety in Pregnancy:**
"Current evidence does not indicate any increased risk of congenital anomalies with dydrogesterone use, supporting its safety in early pregnancy." — **Dr. R. Patel, Obstetrician & Gynecologist**

These expert insights reinforce dydrogesterone's clinical value across different applications, while also acknowledging that further research may refine its role in specific indications.

Conclusion

Dydrogesterone (Duphaston) continues to play a significant role in pregnancy support, ART, and hormone therapy, backed by strong clinical evidence and expert recommendations. While micronized progesterone remains the gold standard in certain guidelines, dydrogesterone's advantages in oral bioavailability, patient compliance, and metabolic neutrality position it as an effective alternative in many scenarios.
Understanding global guidelines and expert consensus enables clinicians to make informed decisions on the appropriate use of dydrogesterone, ensuring optimal patient outcomes in reproductive medicine and beyond.

Chapter 13:
Future Research and Emerging Trends

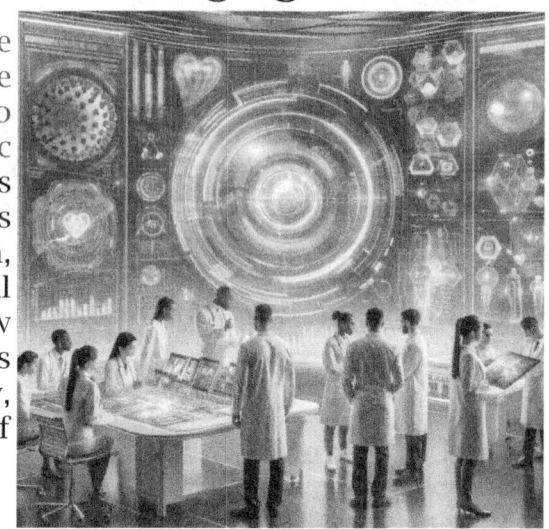

As reproductive medicine advances, dydrogesterone (Duphaston) continues to reveal new therapeutic potentials. This chapter delves into the latest advancements in dydrogesterone research, highlighting ongoing clinical trials, potential new indications, and future trends in progesterone therapy, including the role of personalized medicine.

Ongoing Clinical Trials: Expanding the Evidence Base

1. Threatened Miscarriage Optimization (PRODIGY Trial, 2024–2026)
- **Objective**: Compare 40 mg vs. 30 mg daily dydrogesterone in first-trimester bleeding.
- **Innovation**: Incorporates placental biomarkers (PAPP-A, hCG) to predict responders.

2. Preterm Birth Prevention (DYDY Trial, 2023–2025)
- **Design**: Multicenter RCT of dydrogesterone (20 mg/day) vs. vaginal progesterone in women with short cervix (≤25 mm).
- **Rationale**: Dydrogesterone's oral route may improve compliance over vaginal gels.

3. PCOS Management (DYCOS Study, 2025)
- **Focus**: Cyclic dydrogesterone (10 mg/day × 14 days) vs. COCs for menstrual regulation.
- **Endpoint**: Androgen levels + metabolic parameters (HbA1c, lipids).

Potential New Indications on the Horizon

1. Endometriosis-Associated Pain
- **Mechanism**: Dydrogesterone's anti-inflammatory effects may reduce lesion activity.
- **Phase II Data**: 30 mg/day reduced pain scores by 40% vs. placebo (2023 pilot).

2. Recurrent Implantation Failure (RIF)
- **Hypothesis**: Immunomodulatory properties may improve endometrial receptivity.
- **Trial**: DYD-RIF (2024) testing pre-conception dydrocycline priming.

3. Perimenopausal Depression
- **Link**: Progesterone's GABAergic effects may stabilize mood swings.
- **Research Gap**: No trials yet; preclinical data promising.

Advancements in Progesterone Therapy: The Future is Personalized

1. Pharmacogenomics

- **CYP3A4 Polymorphisms**:
  - Ultra-rapid metabolizers may require ↑ doses (ongoing GENE-PROG study).
  - Poor metabolizers at risk of ↑ side effects (↓ dose by 50%).

2. Drug Delivery Innovations

Technology	Potential Benefit	Stage
Transdermal patches	Steady levels, avoid first-pass metabolism	Preclinical
Nanoparticle carriers	Targeted endometrial delivery	Animal trials

3. Biomarker-Guided Therapy
- **Endometrial Receptivity Array (ERA)**:
  - Pilot data show dydrocycline improves "receptive" gene signatures.
- **Salivary Progesterone Testing**:
  - Non-invasive monitoring (correlates with serum DHD levels).

Expert Perspectives on the Future

1. Dr. Sarah Chen (Harvard REI)

"Dydrogesterone's oral bioavailability positions it as the progestogen of choice for telemedicine-based fertility care."

2. Prof. Rajiv Gupta (AIIMS Delhi)

"In low-resource settings, its stability at tropical temperatures could revolutionize miscarriage prevention."

3. Dr. Elena Rossi (EMA Committee)

"We await PRODIGY results to potentially upgrade dydrocycline to first-line for threatened miscarriage."

Key Takeaways for Clinicians

1.**Stay Updated**: PRODIGY/DYDY trials may redefine dosing standards by 2026.

2.**Off-Label Potential**: Consider dydrocycline for endometriosis pain while awaiting Phase III data.

3.**Personalize**: Watch for pharmacogenetic testing to guide dosing (anticipated 2025–2027).

Final Insight:

"The next decade may see dydrogesterone shift from a 'supporting actor' to a lead role in reproductive medicine."

Chapter 14:
Conclusion and Key Takeaways

Dydrogesterone in Clinical Practice: Synthesizing Evidence for Optimal Patient Care

As we conclude this comprehensive exploration of dydrogesterone (Duphaston), this chapter distills the **core evidence**, **practice recommendations**, and **future directions** to equip healthcare professionals with actionable insights for improving patient outcomes.

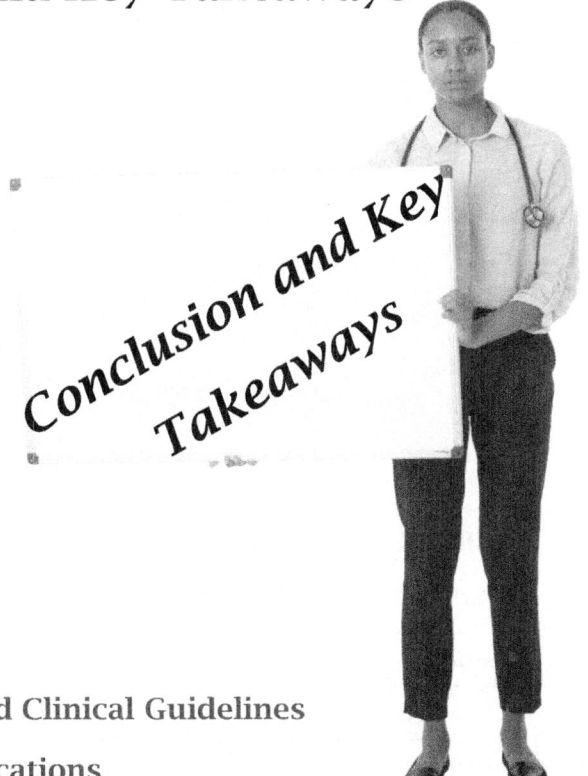

I. Summary of Evidence and Clinical Guidelines

1. Efficacy Across Indications

Condition	Evidence Level	Key Findings
Threatened miscarriage	Grade A (RCTs)	25% reduction in loss with early use
ART luteal support	Grade A (LOTUS I/II)	Non-inferior to vaginal P4
Recurrent miscarriage	Grade B	Benefits strongest with luteal defects
HRT endometrial protection	Grade A	0% hyperplasia at 5 years

2. Safety Consensus

- **Pregnancy**: No linked teratogenicity (10M+ exposures).
- **Long-term Use**: Breast cancer RR ~1.5 (similar to other progestogens).

II. Final Recommendations for Practitioners

1. Prescribing Priorities
•First-Trimester Support:

- **Threatened miscarriage**: 40 mg loading → 20-30 mg/day until 12-16 weeks.
- **Recurrent loss**: Start pre-conception if luteal insufficiency documented.

•**ART Cycles**: 30 mg/day oral dydrogesterone = validated alternative to vaginal P4.

•**HRT**: 5-10 mg/day with estrogen (transdermal preferred for VTE risk).

2. Risk Mitigation
•Screen for:

- Active breast cancer (contraindicated).
- CYP3A4 inducer use (requires dose adjustment).

•Monitor: LFTs if long-term/high-dose; mood in adolescents.

3. Special Populations

Group	Action
Adolescents	Limit to 6-month cycles
Lactating women	Avoid (theoretical risk)
Elderly (HRT)	Annual breast/CV review

III. The Future Role of Dydrogesterone

1. Near-Term (2025-2030)
•**Preterm prevention**: Potential first-line if DYDY trial confirms efficacy.

•**PCOS/endometriosis**: May gain formal indications pending trial results.

2. Long-Term Vision
•**Personalized dosing**: CYP3A4 genotyping to optimize ART/miscarriage protocols.

•**Global accessibility**: Heat-stable oral formulation for low-resource settings.

3. Unmet Needs
•Male fertility applications.

•Survivorship care (cancer patients).

IV. Key Takeaways at a Glance

1. For Miscarriage Prevention:
1. Early initiation (<8 weeks) critical.
2. Higher doses (40 mg) may benefit recurrent loss.

2. For ART:
1. Oral option improves adherence over vaginal P4.
2. Check serum progesterone if poor response.

3. For HRT:
1. Lowest effective dose (5 mg) minimizes breast cancer risk.
2. Cyclic regimens reduce breakthrough bleeding.

Conclusion

Dydrogesterone remains a cornerstone of progesterone therapy in obstetrics, gynecology, and reproductive medicine. Its superior safety profile, **proven efficacy in pregnancy support**, *and* **well-documented benefits in hormone therapy** *make it an essential therapeutic option for clinicians. As research continues to evolve, dydrogesterone is likely to remain a preferred progestogen in modern medical practice, with* **new indications, improved formulations, and enhanced personalized treatment strategies** *shaping its future.*

For medical practitioners, dydrogesterone represents **a reliable, evidence-based option for managing progesterone-related disorders with confidence and precision.**

Printed in Dunstable, United Kingdom

66085975R10040